COLORING BOOK FOR TEENS

Positive Affirmations For Teens With Anxiety

"You can't always control what goes on outside.
But you can always control what goes on inside."
Wayne Dyer

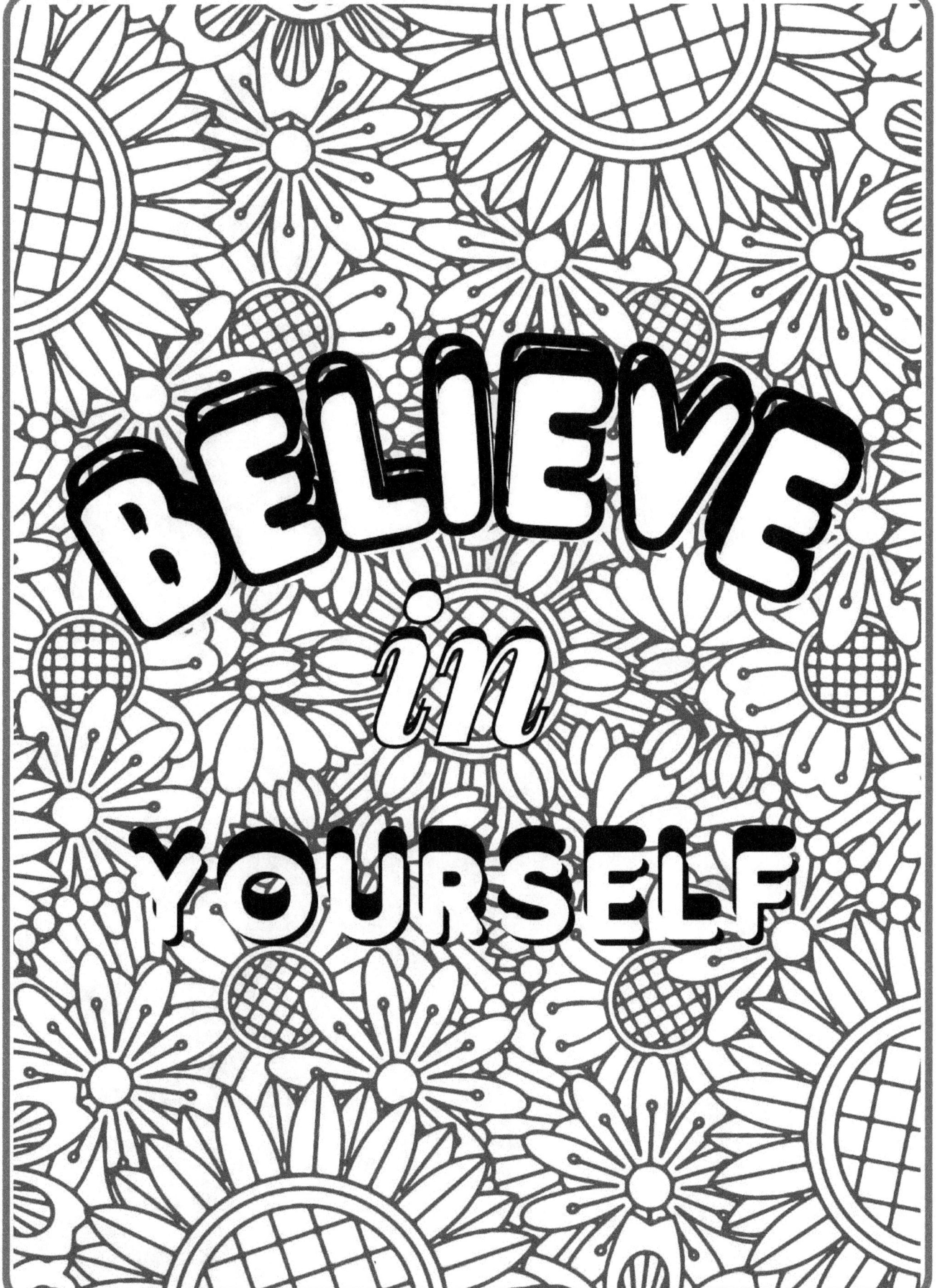
BELIEVE
in
YOURSELF

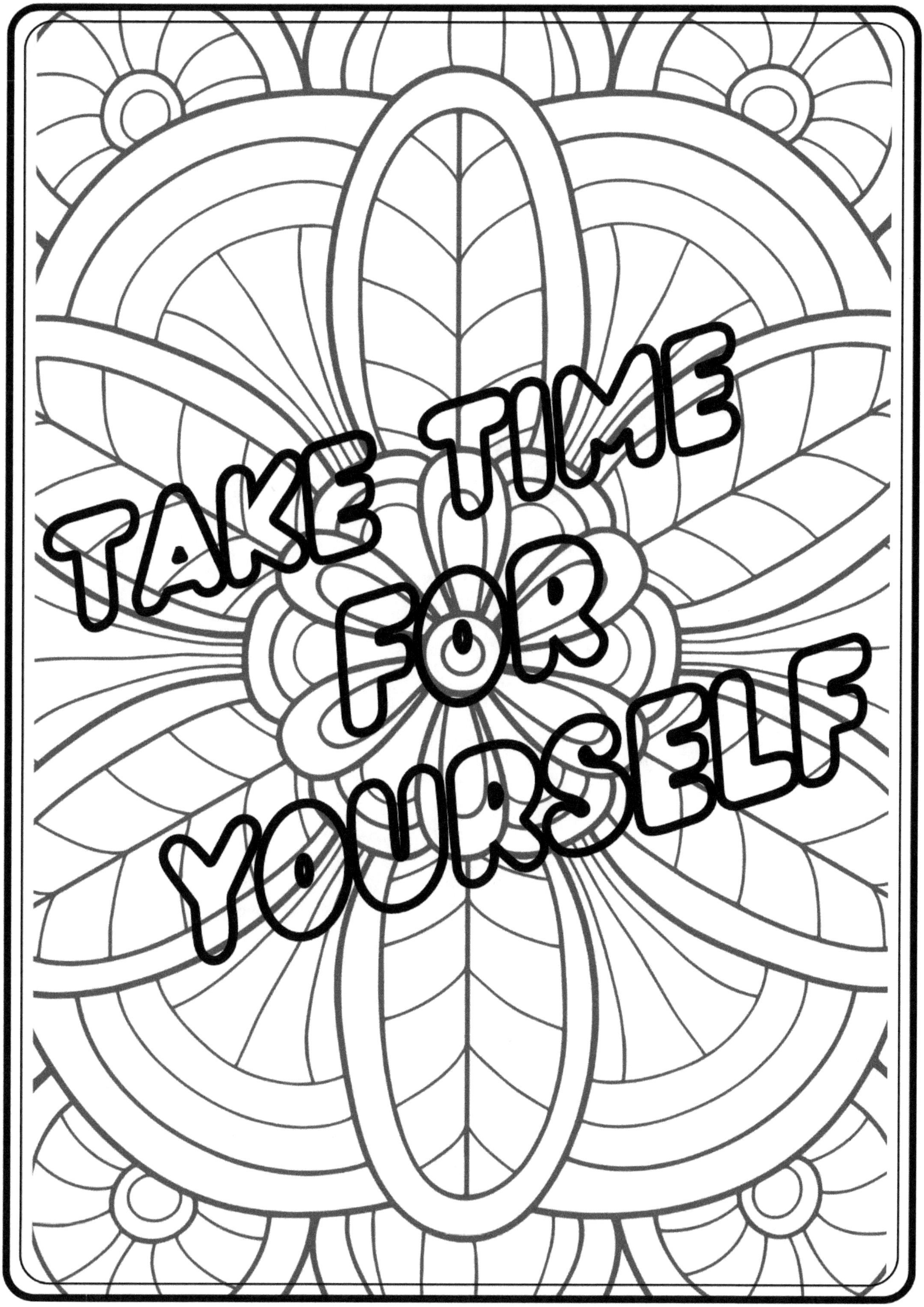
TAKE TIME
FOR
YOURSELF

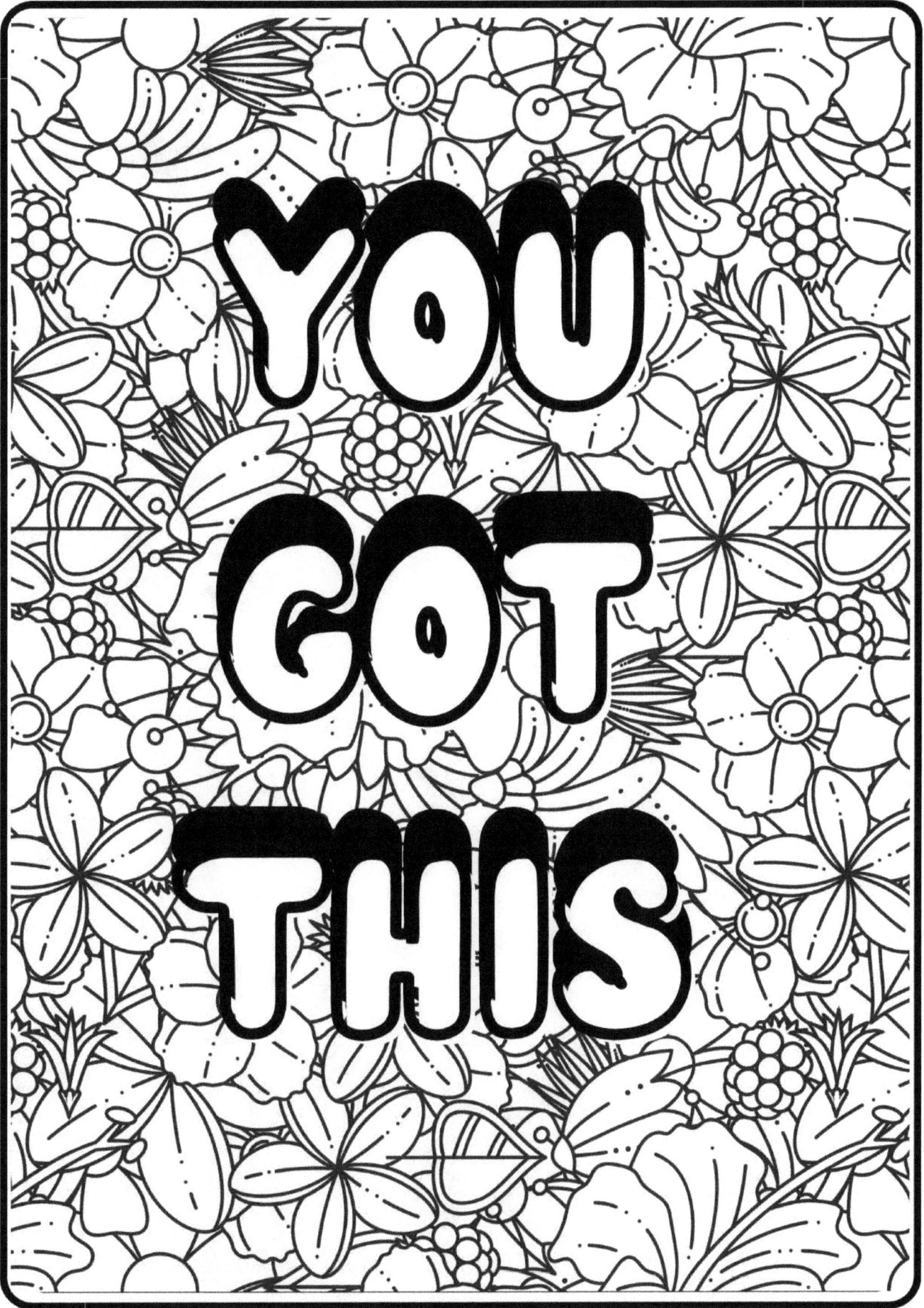

GOOD VIBES ONLY

IT'S OKAY to not be okay

ALL THINGS ARE POSSIBLE IF YOU BELIEVE

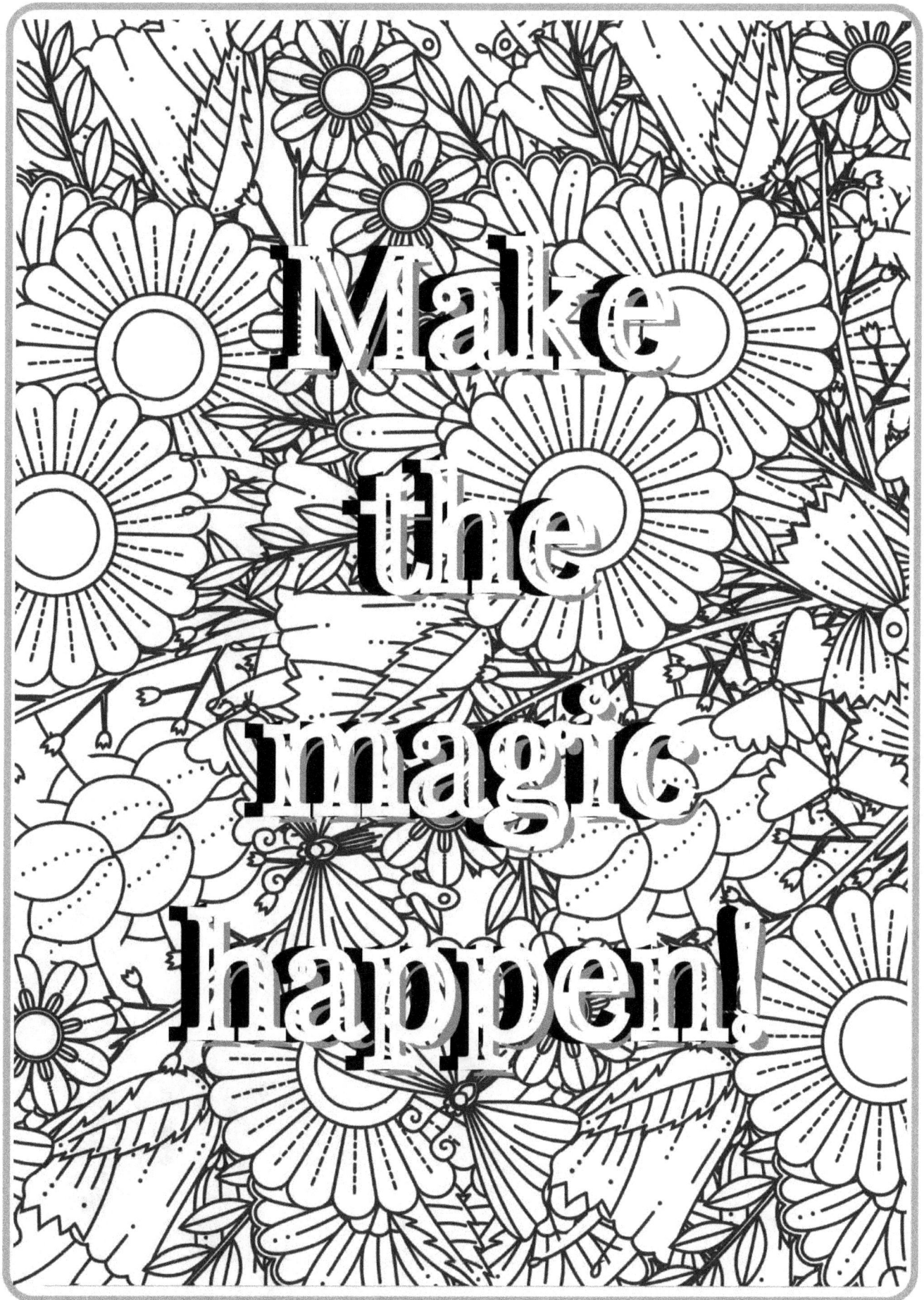

Make the magic happen!

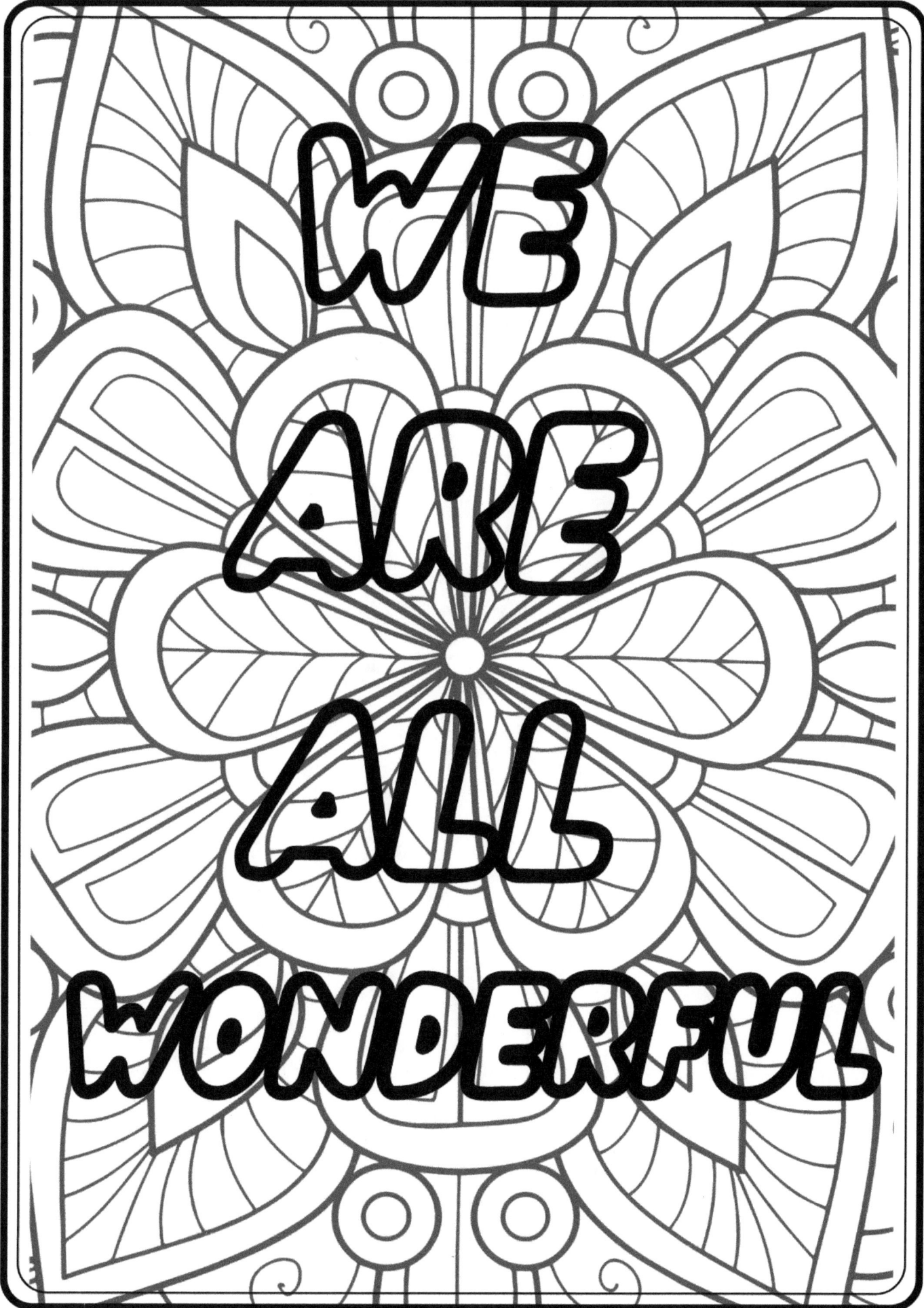

WE ARE ALL WONDERFUL

Be brave
Be bold
Be you

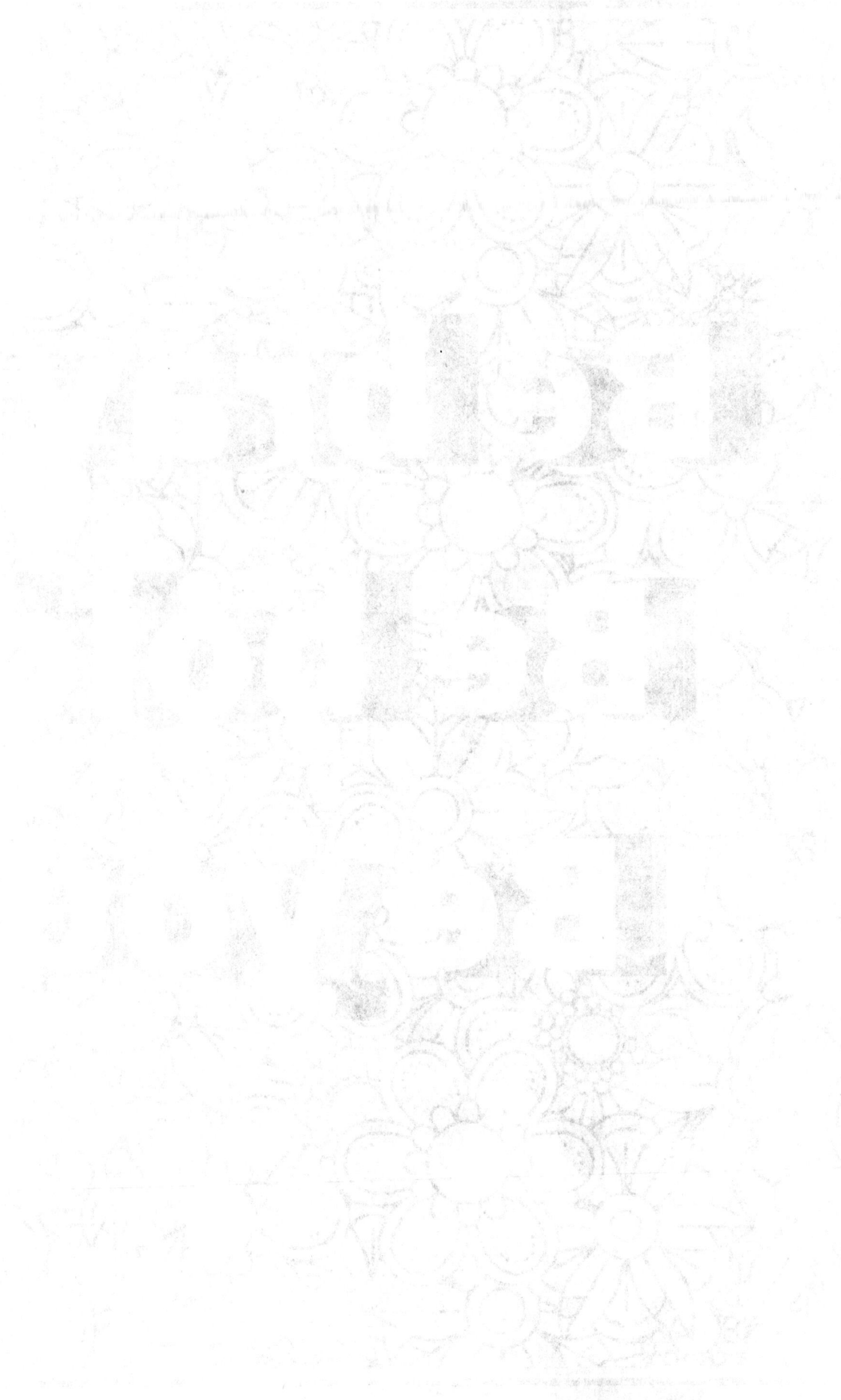

DREAM
BELIEVE
ACHIEVE

IT'S NEVER IMPOSSIBLE JUST TRY

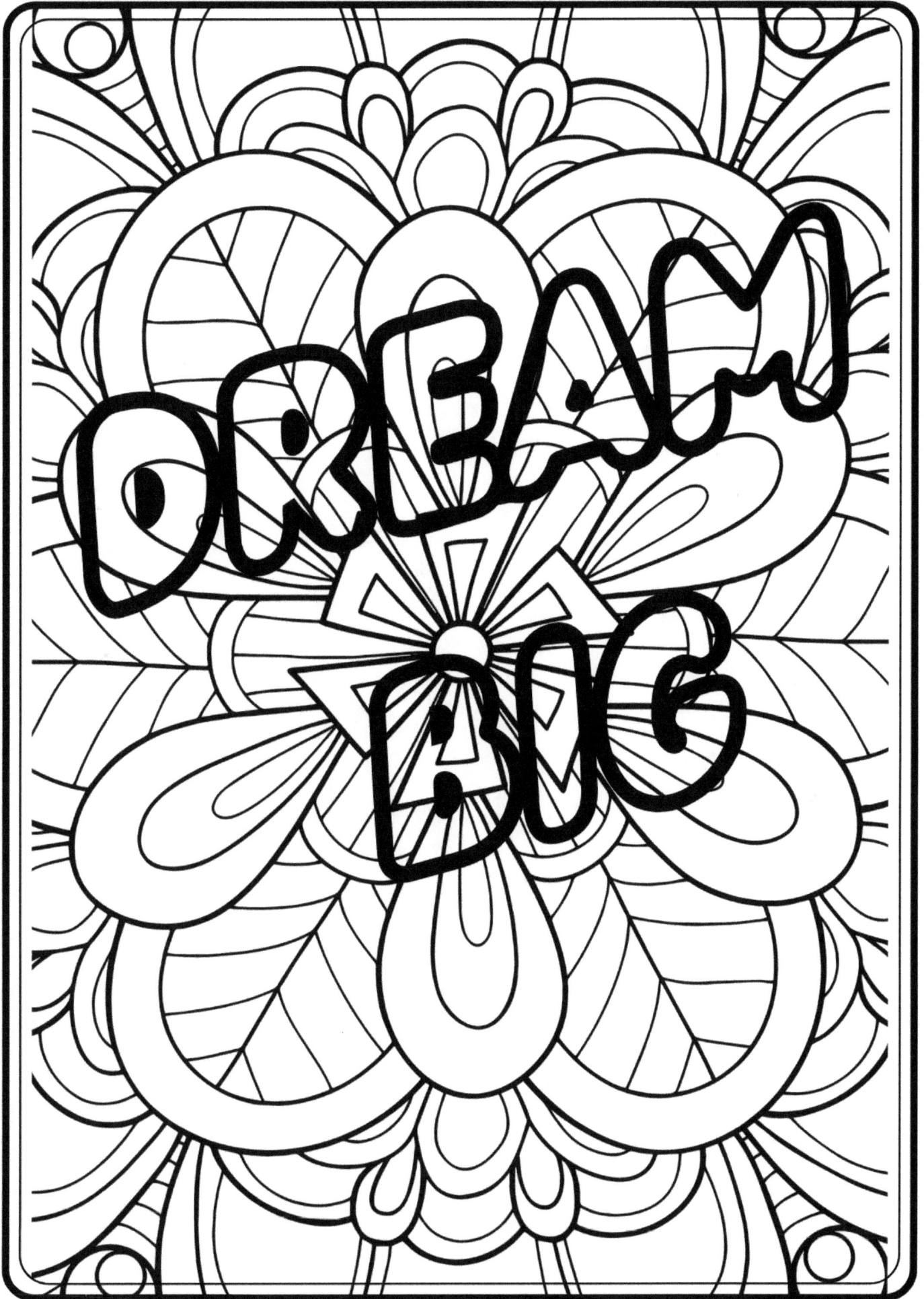

BE A TRUE BADASS

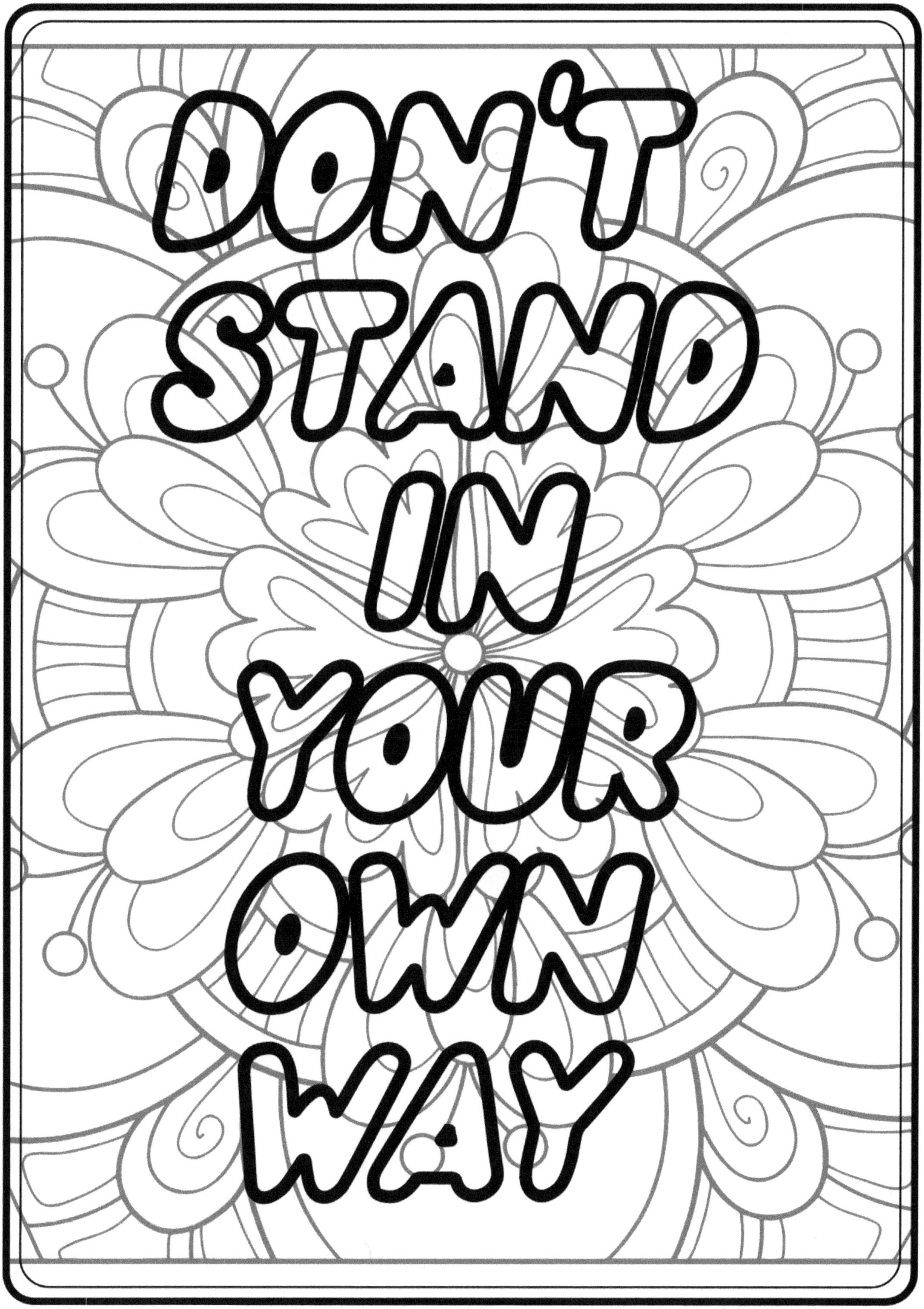
DON'T
STAND
IN
YOUR
OWN
WAY

Find joy in the little things

TAKE A DEEP BREATH AND TRY AGAIN

YOU ARE
POWER
BEAUTIFUL
BRILLIANT

MAKE YOURSELF SEEN AND HEARD

Life is what you make it. Make it a good one

FUELED BY HAPPY THOUGHTS

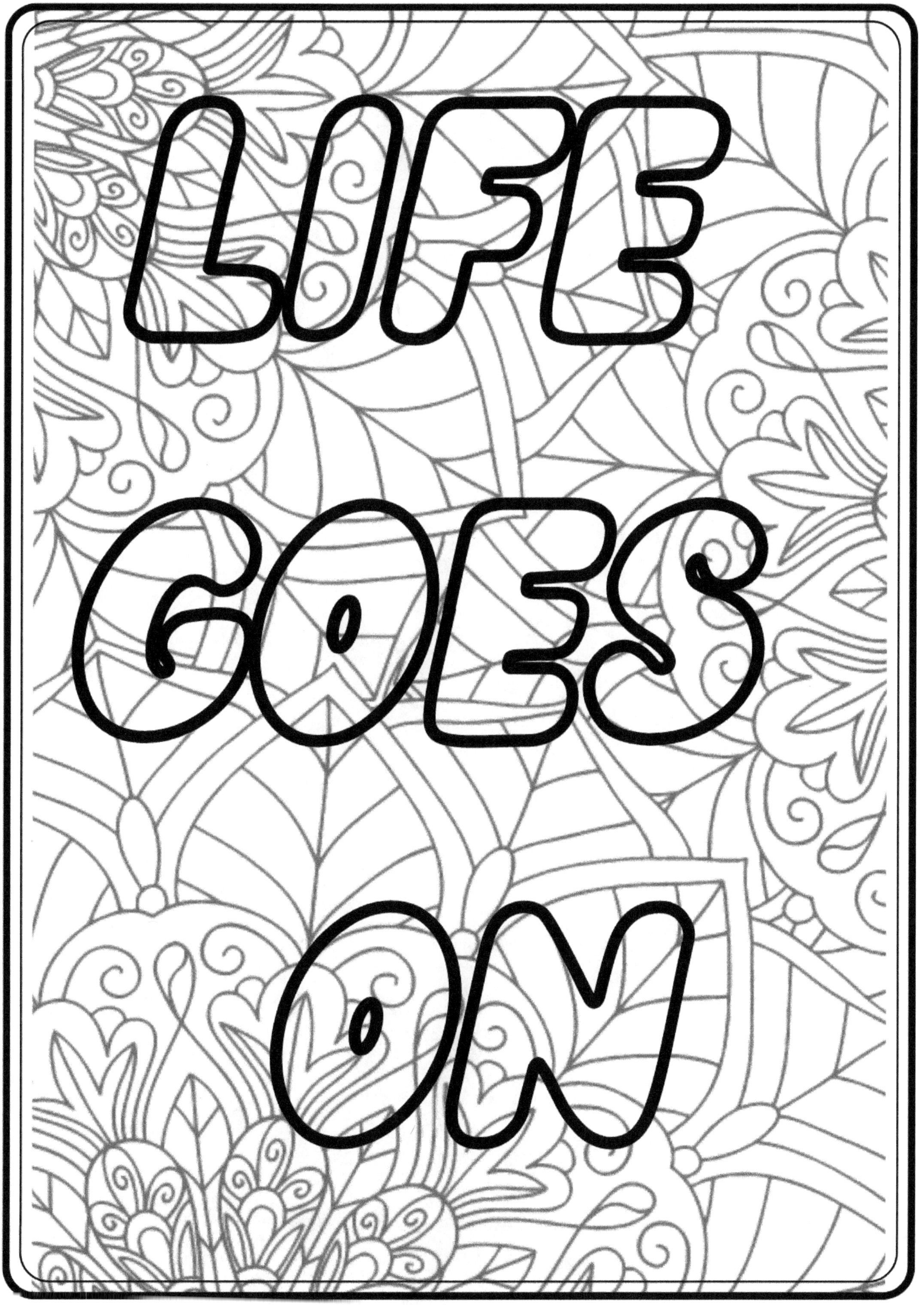
LIFE
GOES
ON

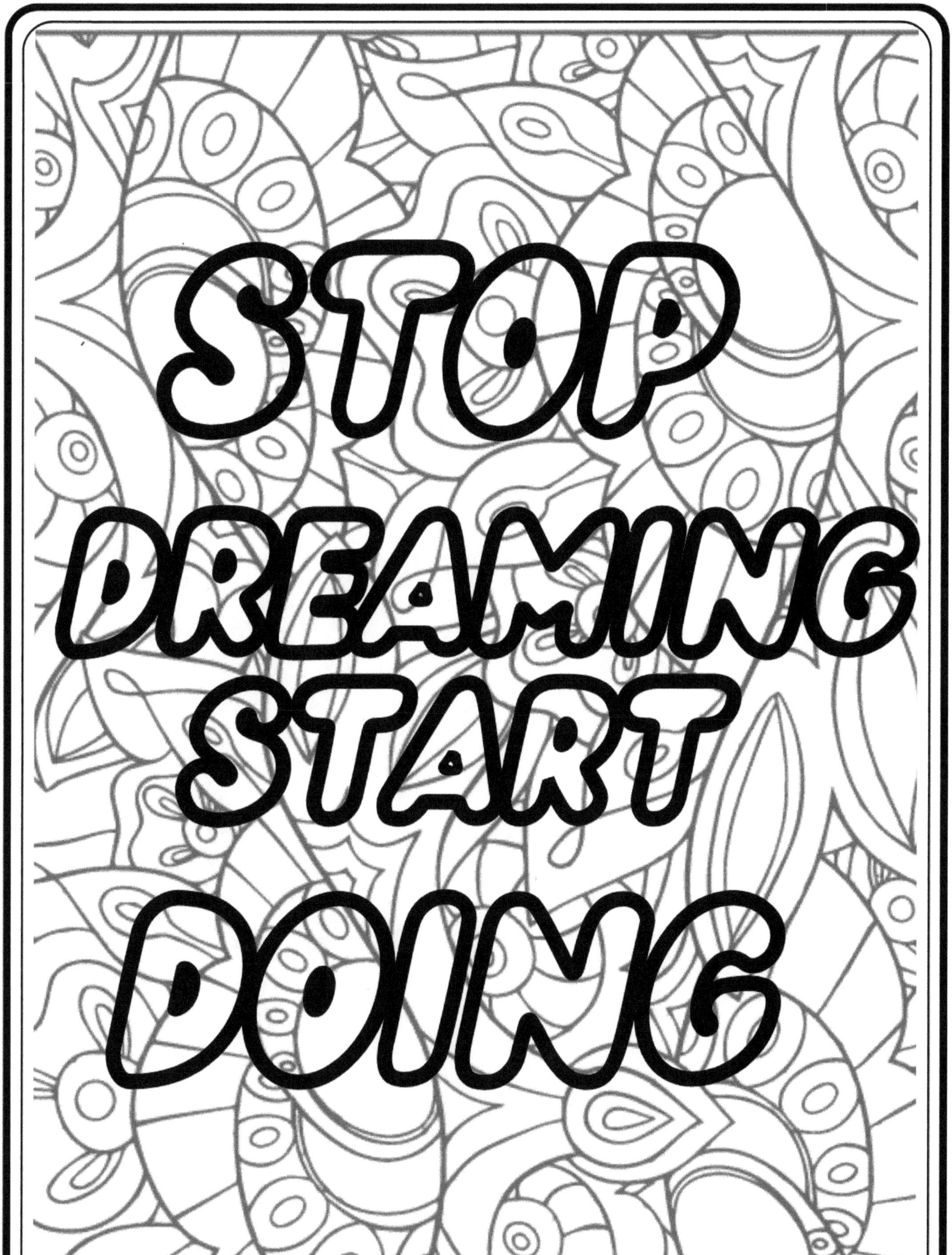
STOP
DREAMING
START
DOING

YOU'RE FREE TO BE DIFFERENT

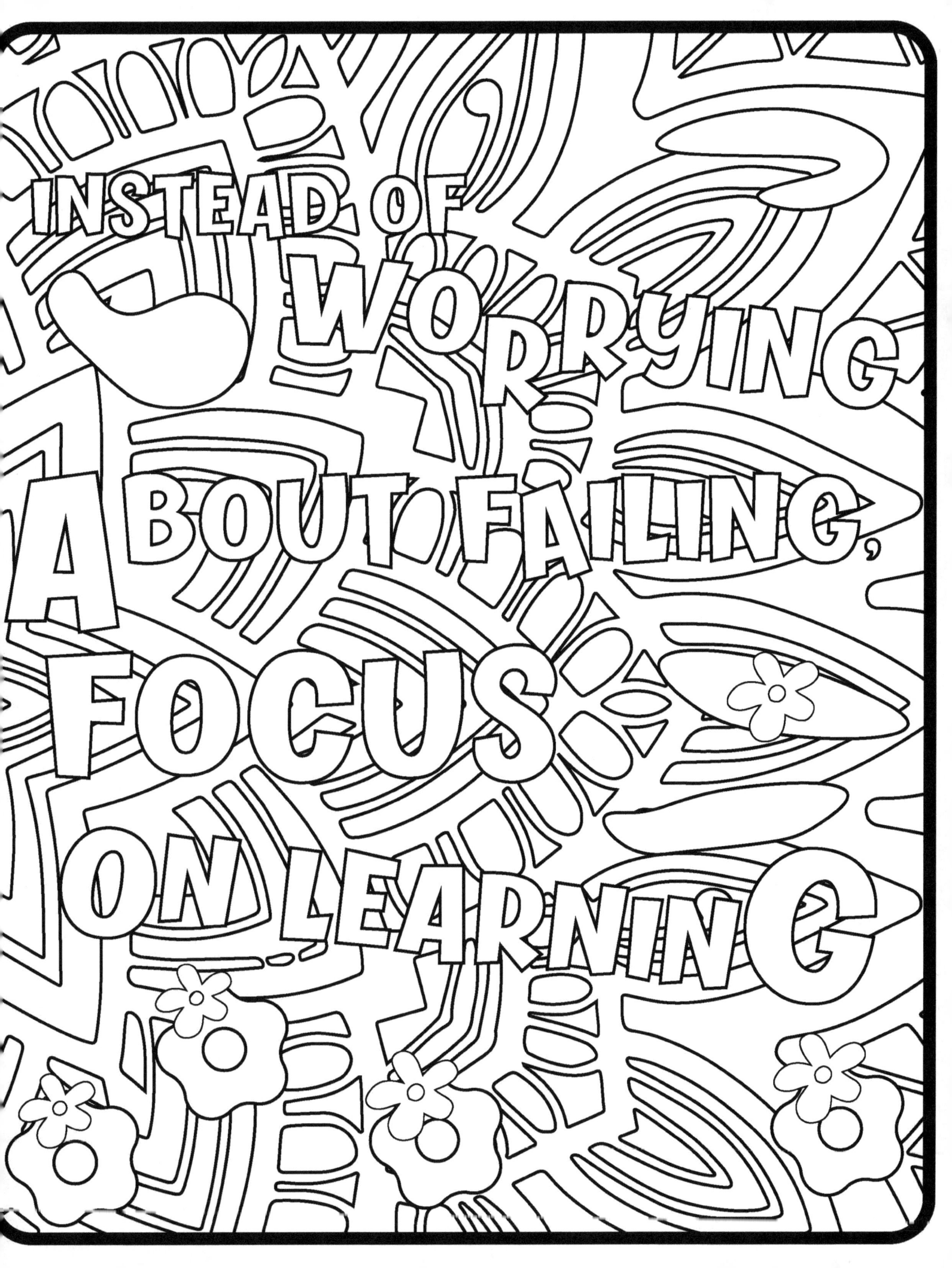

INSTEAD OF WORRYING ABOUT FAILING, FOCUS ON LEARNING

IT'S OKAY TO TAKE A BREAK

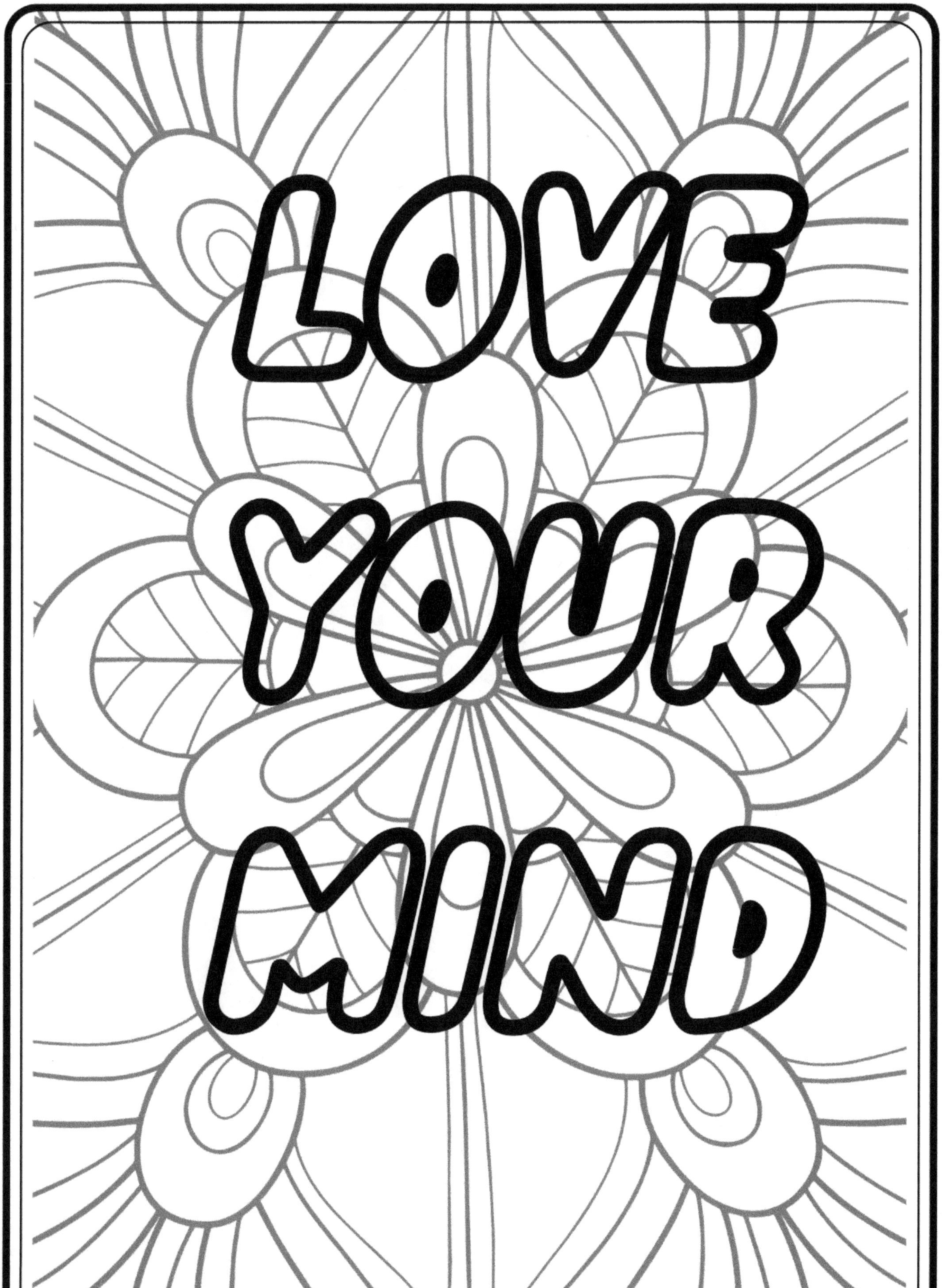
LOVE
YOUR
MIND

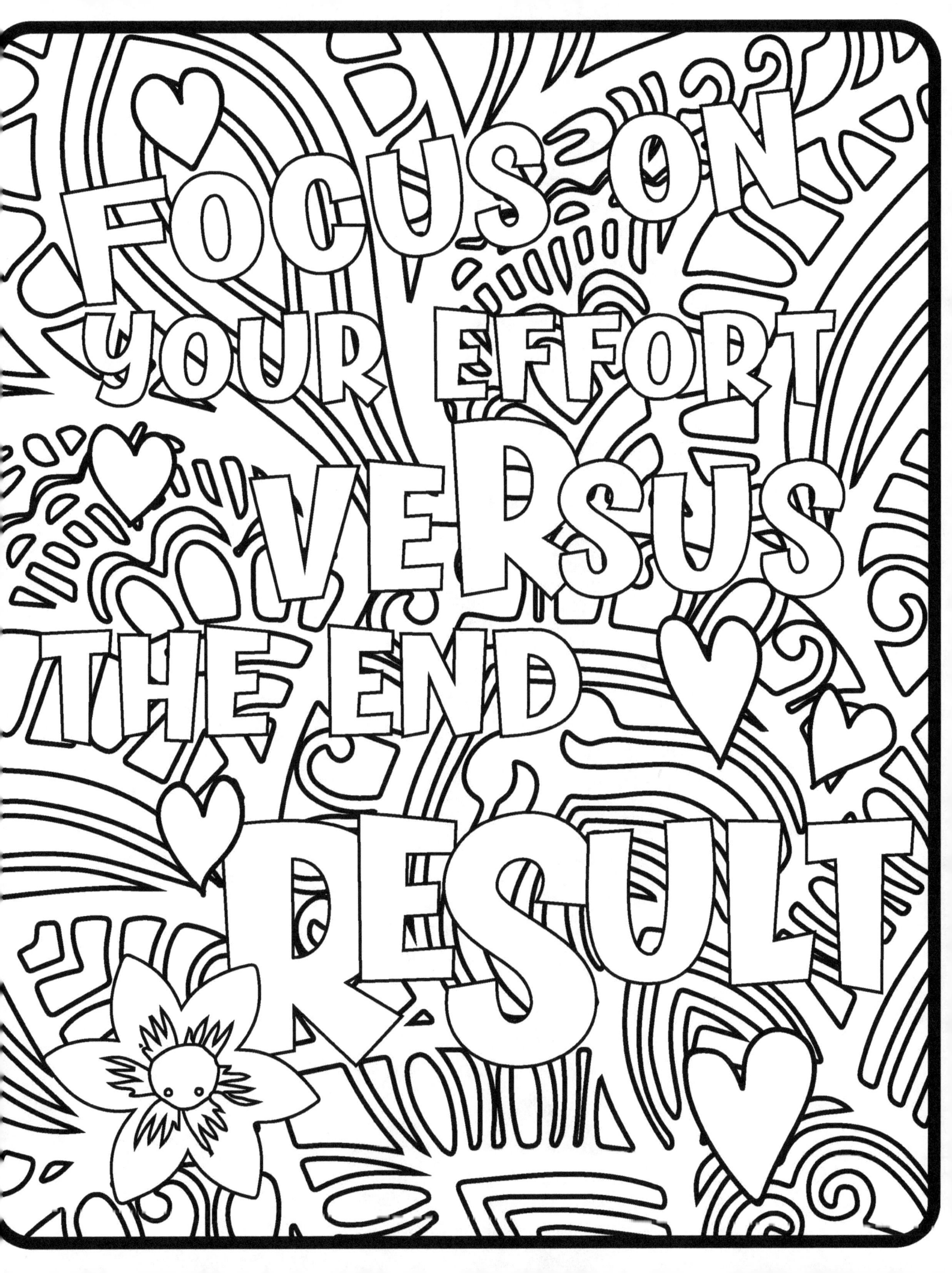

FOCUS ON YOUR EFFORT VERSUS THE END RESULT

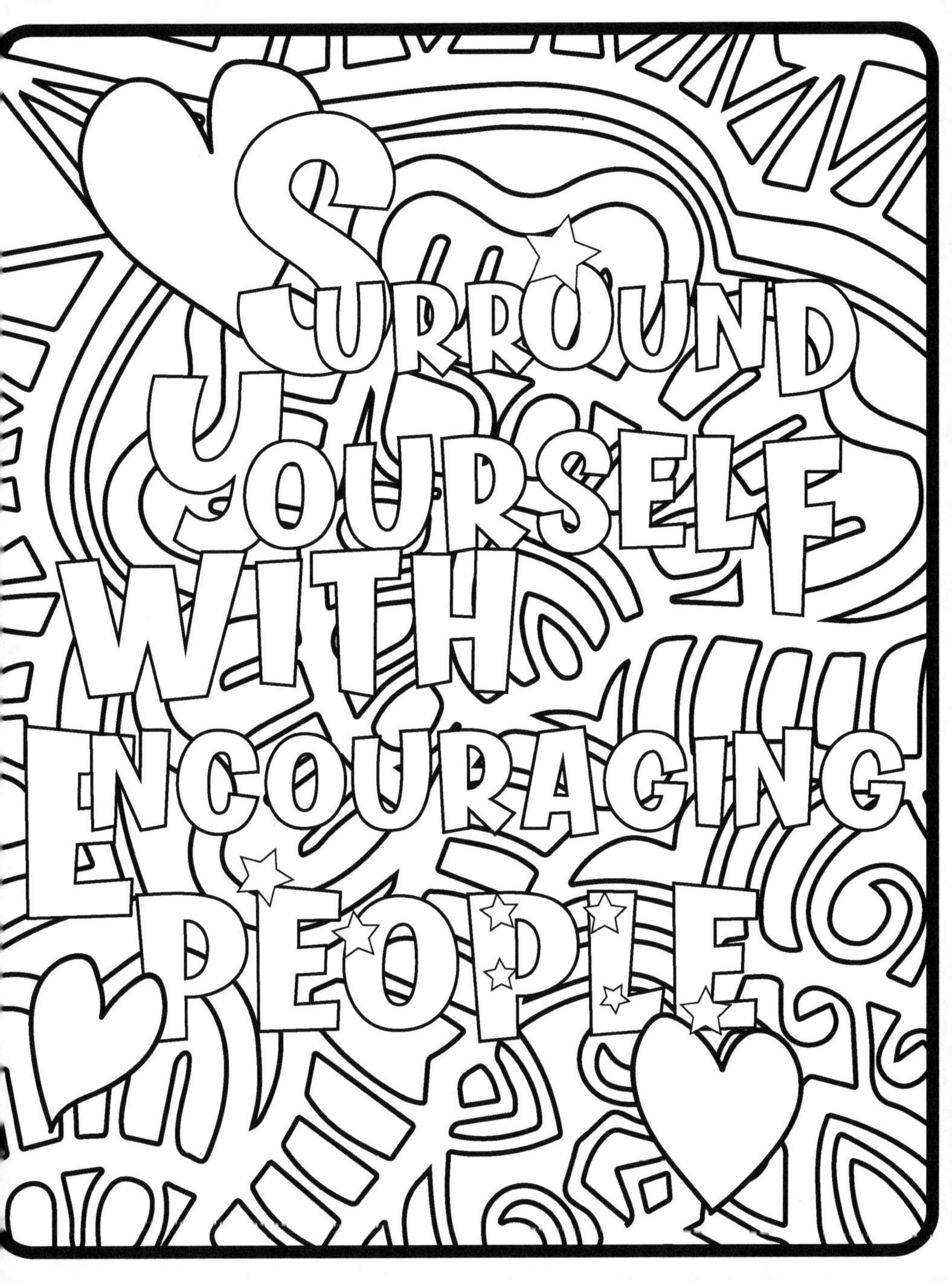

SURROUND YOURSELF WITH ENCOURAGING PEOPLE

SHARE YOUR MINDSET WITH WORK THEM

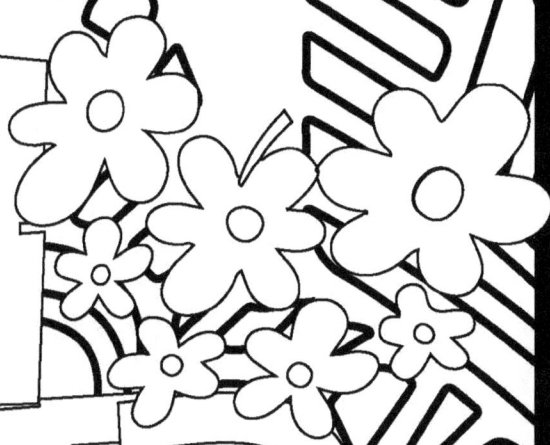

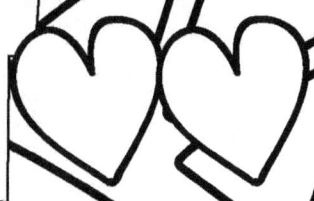

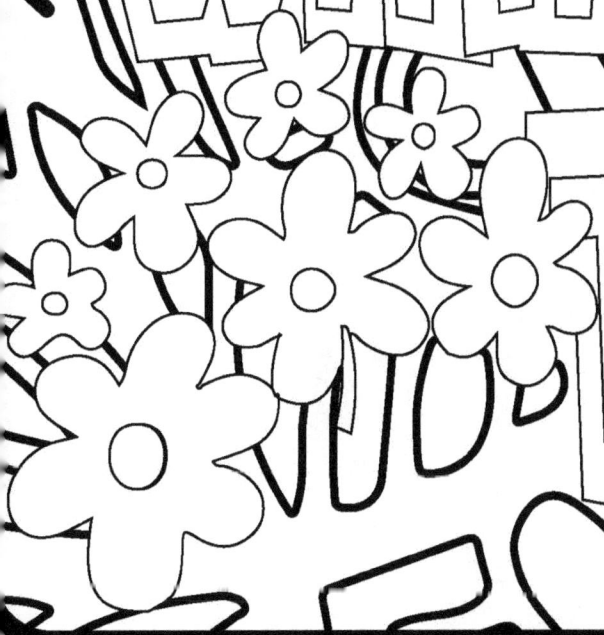

ACCCEPT YOUR IMPERFECTIONS

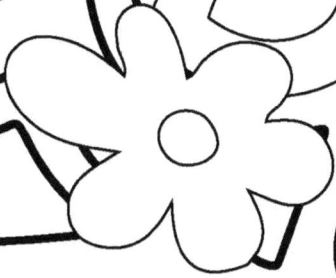

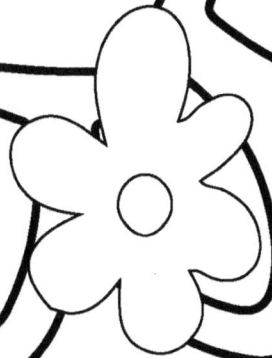

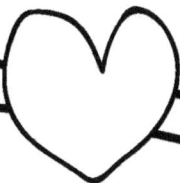

BELIEVE CHANGE AND IMPROVEMENT ARE POSSIBLE

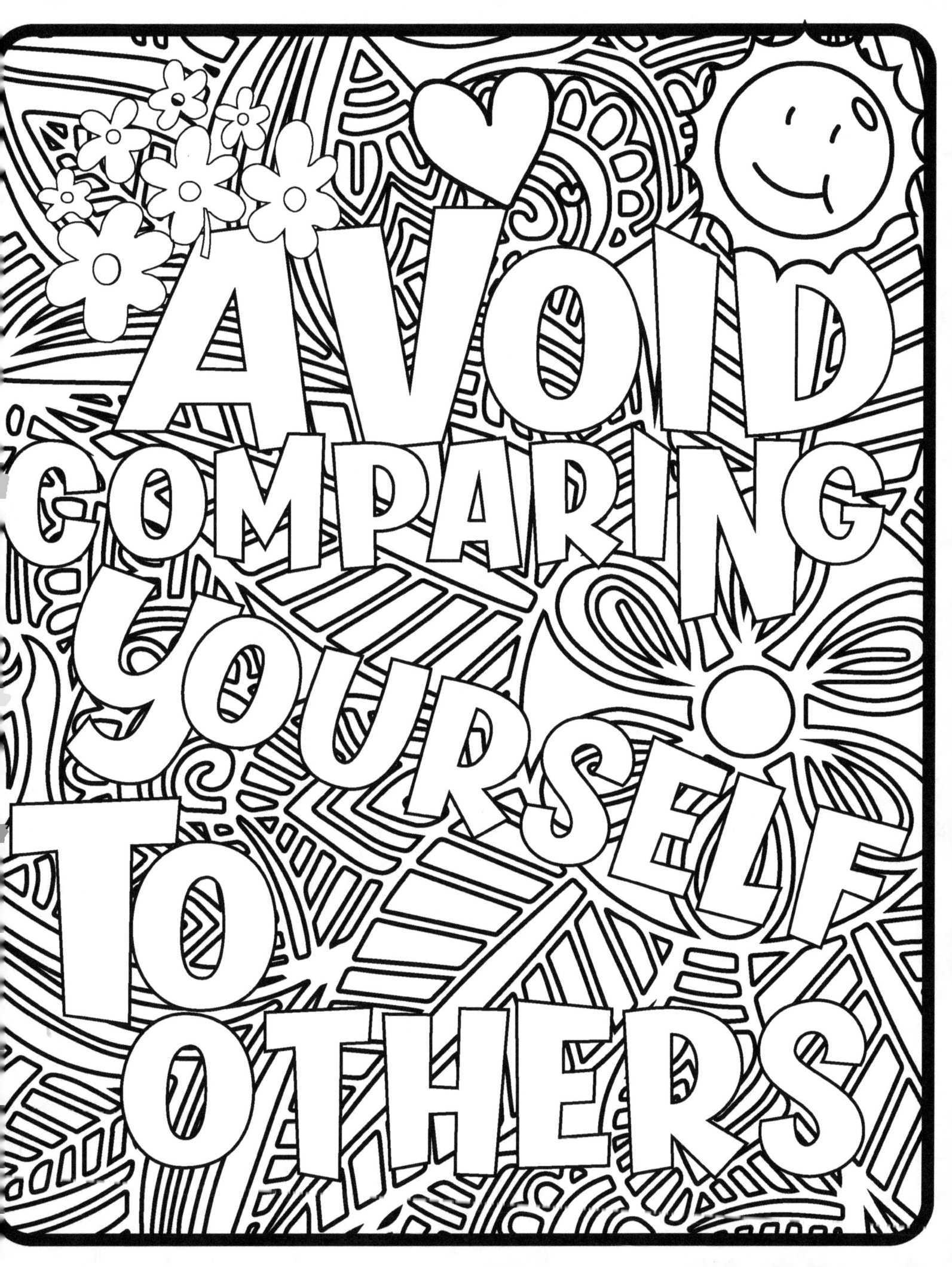

AVOID COMPARING YOURSELF TO OTHERS

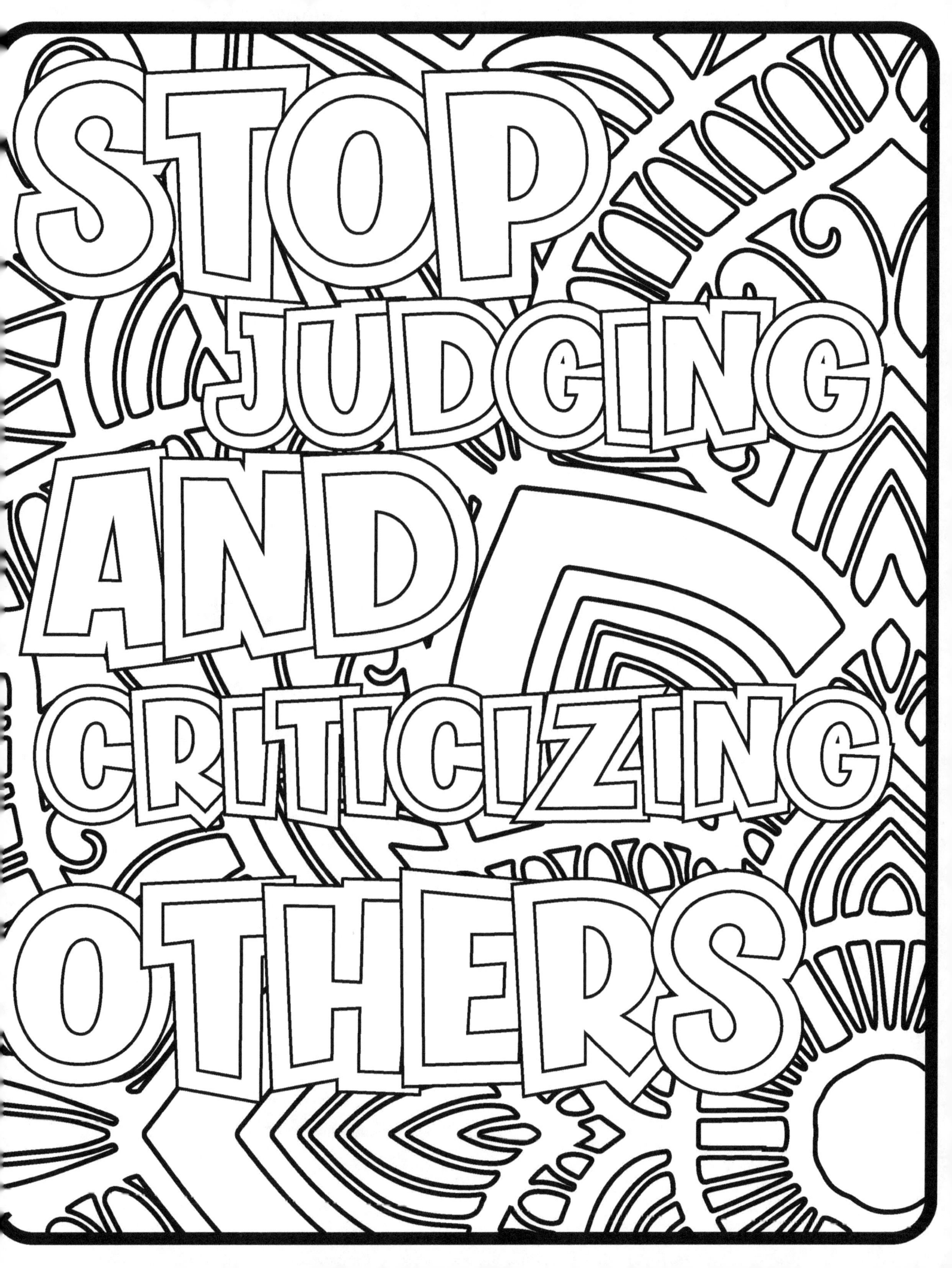

STOP JUDGING AND CRITICIZING OTHERS

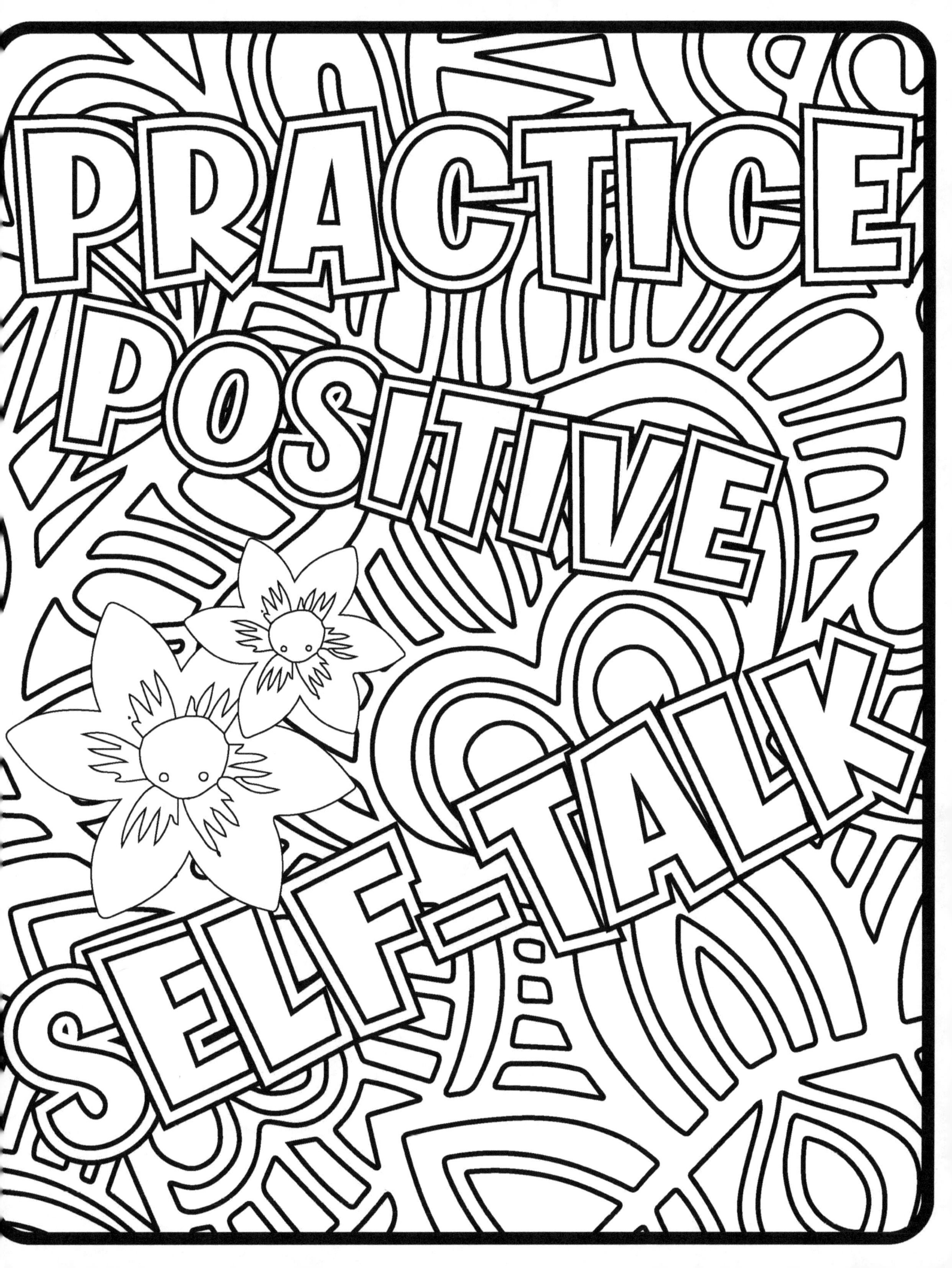

CELEBRATE OTHERS' SUCCESSES

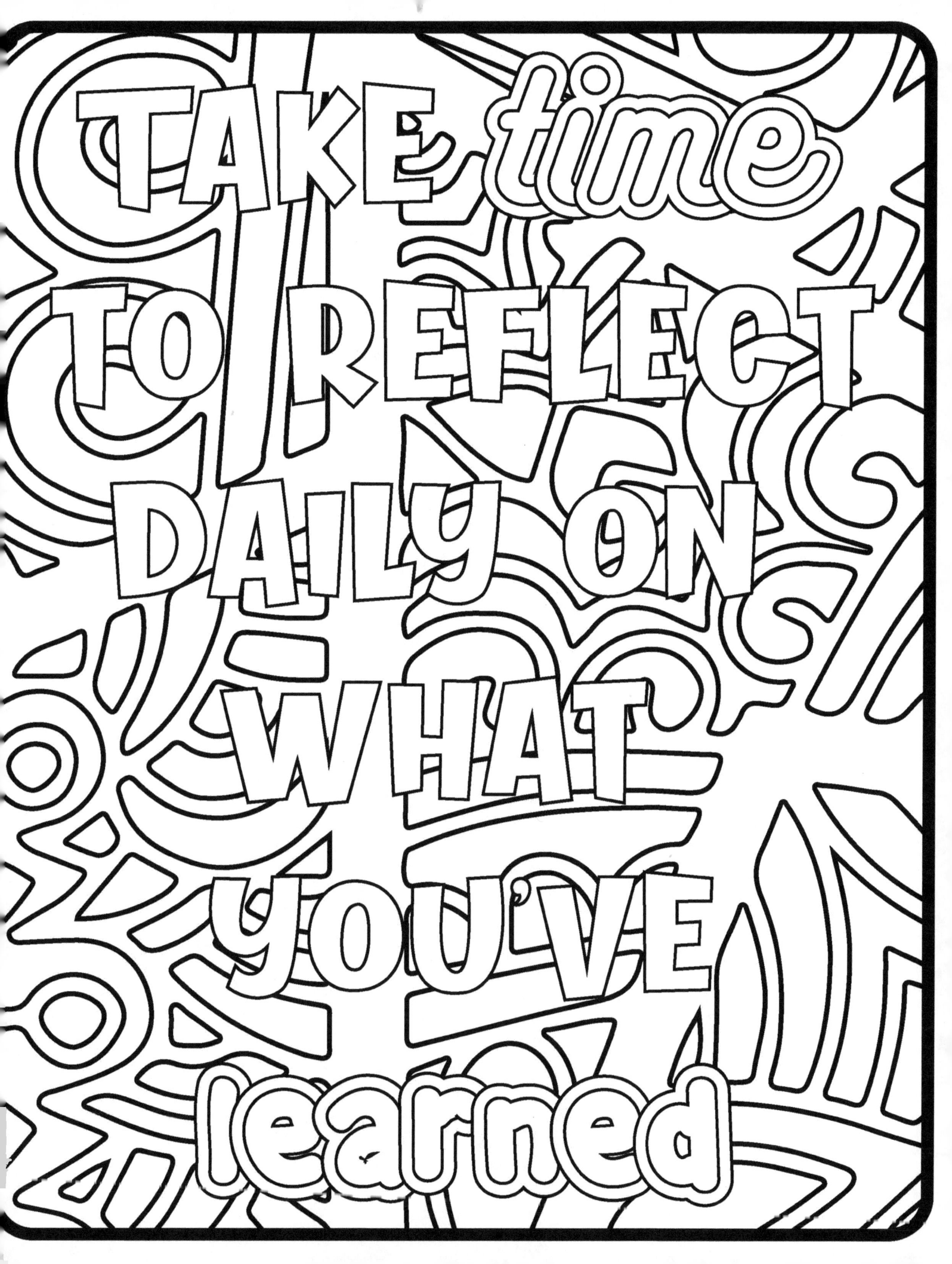

Take time to reflect daily on what you've learned

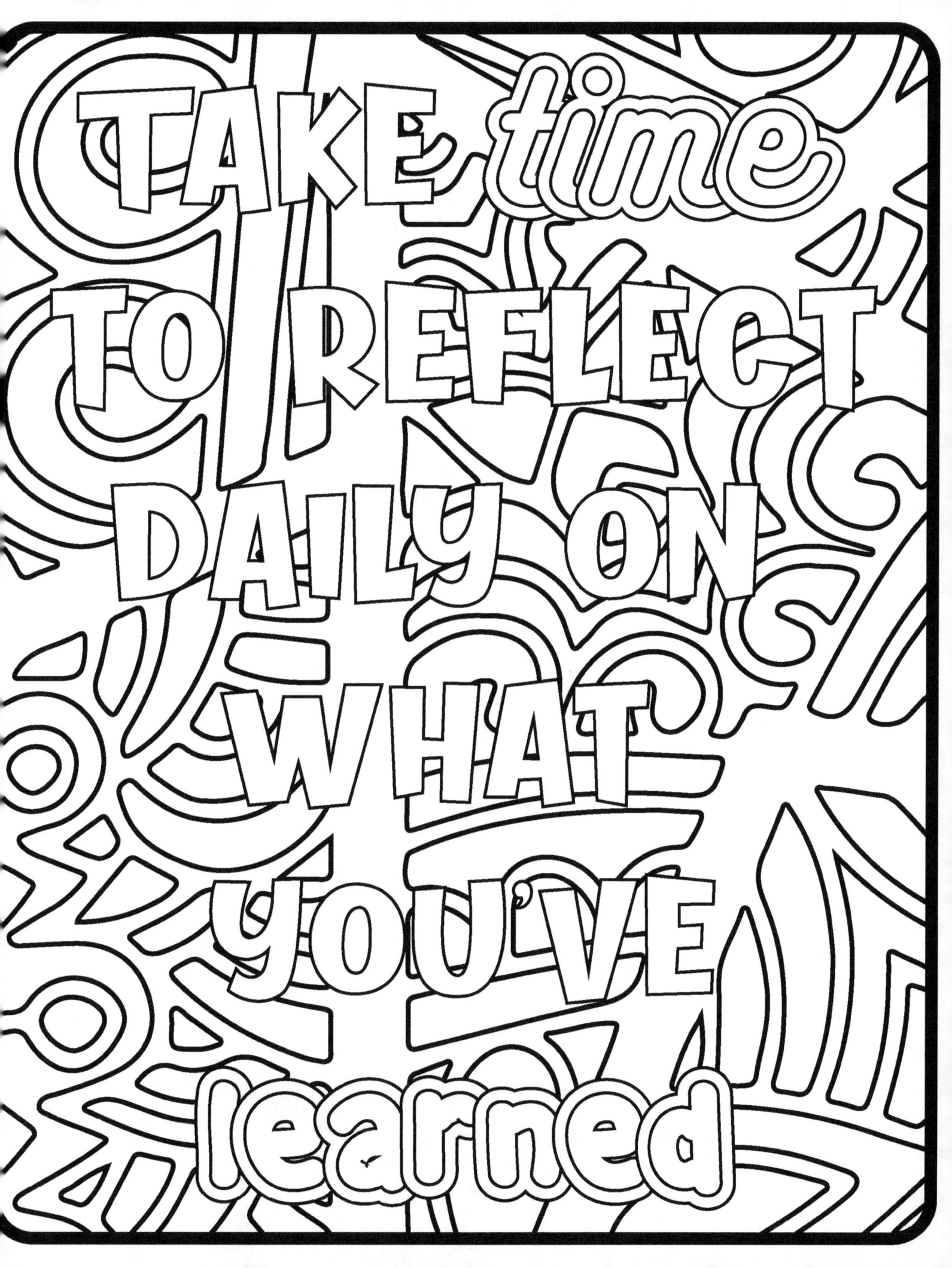

TAKE time TO REFLECT DAILY ON WHAT YOU'VE learned

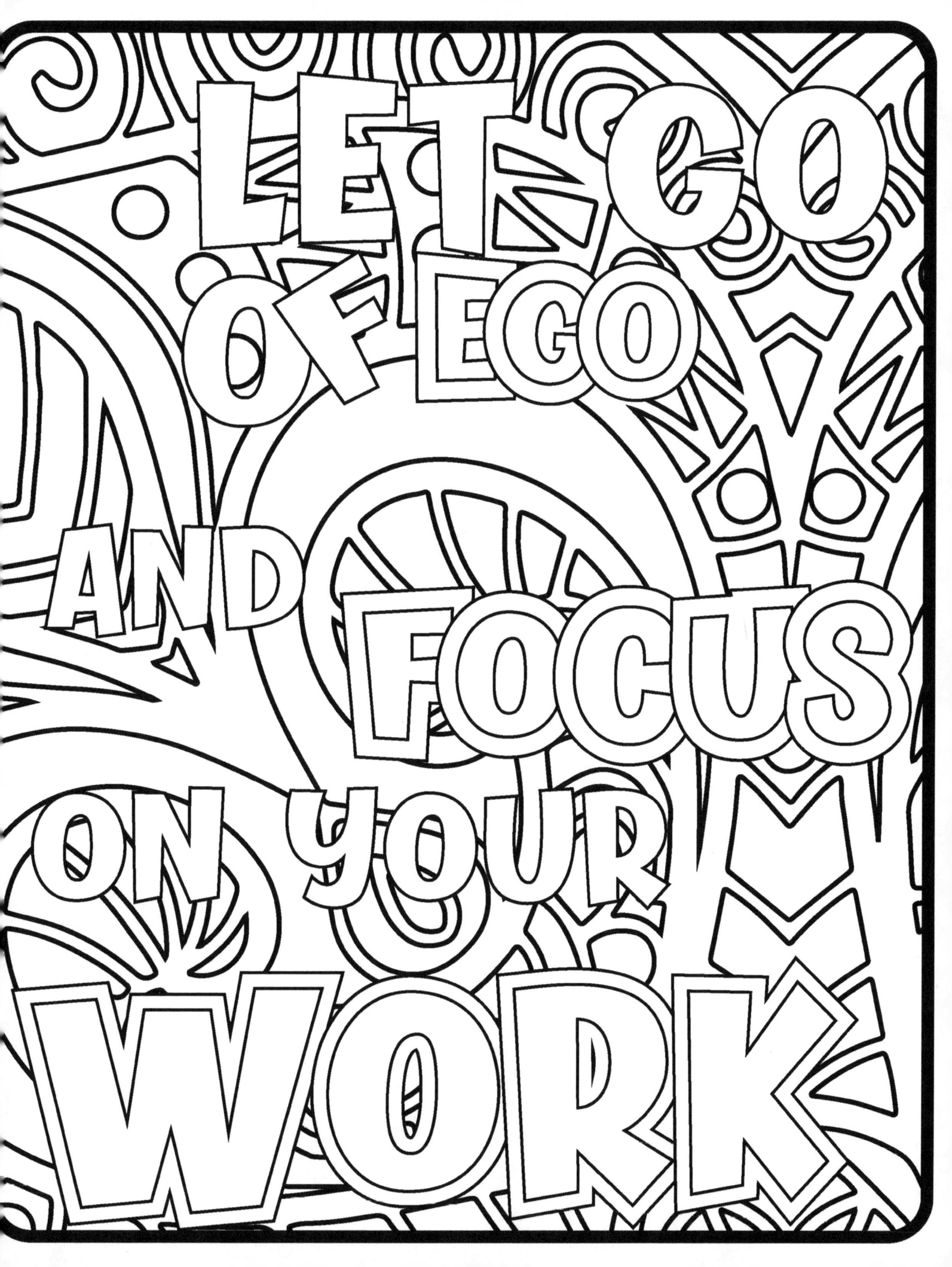
LET GO OF EGO AND FOCUS ON YOUR WORK

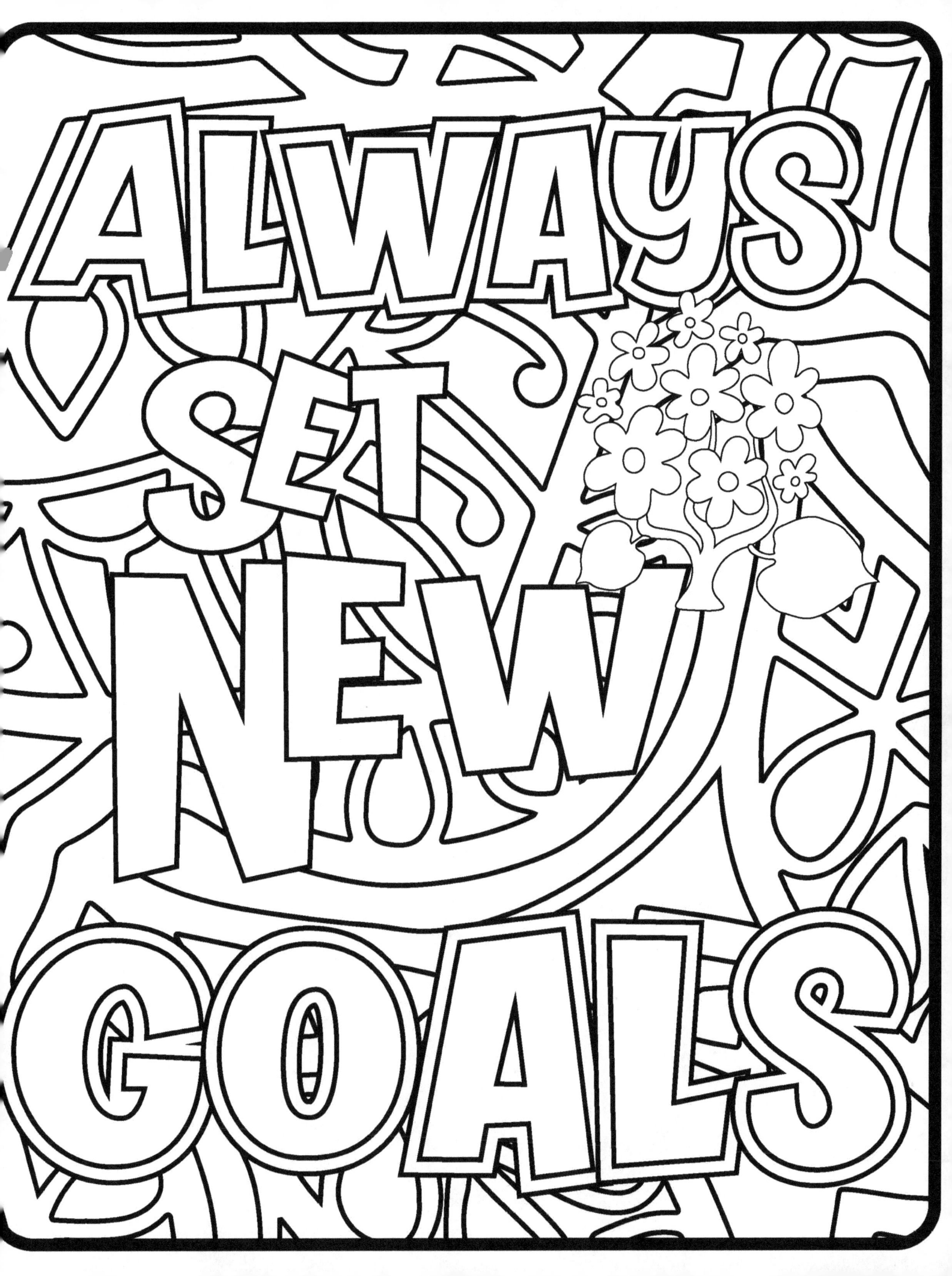

ALWAYS SET NEW GOALS

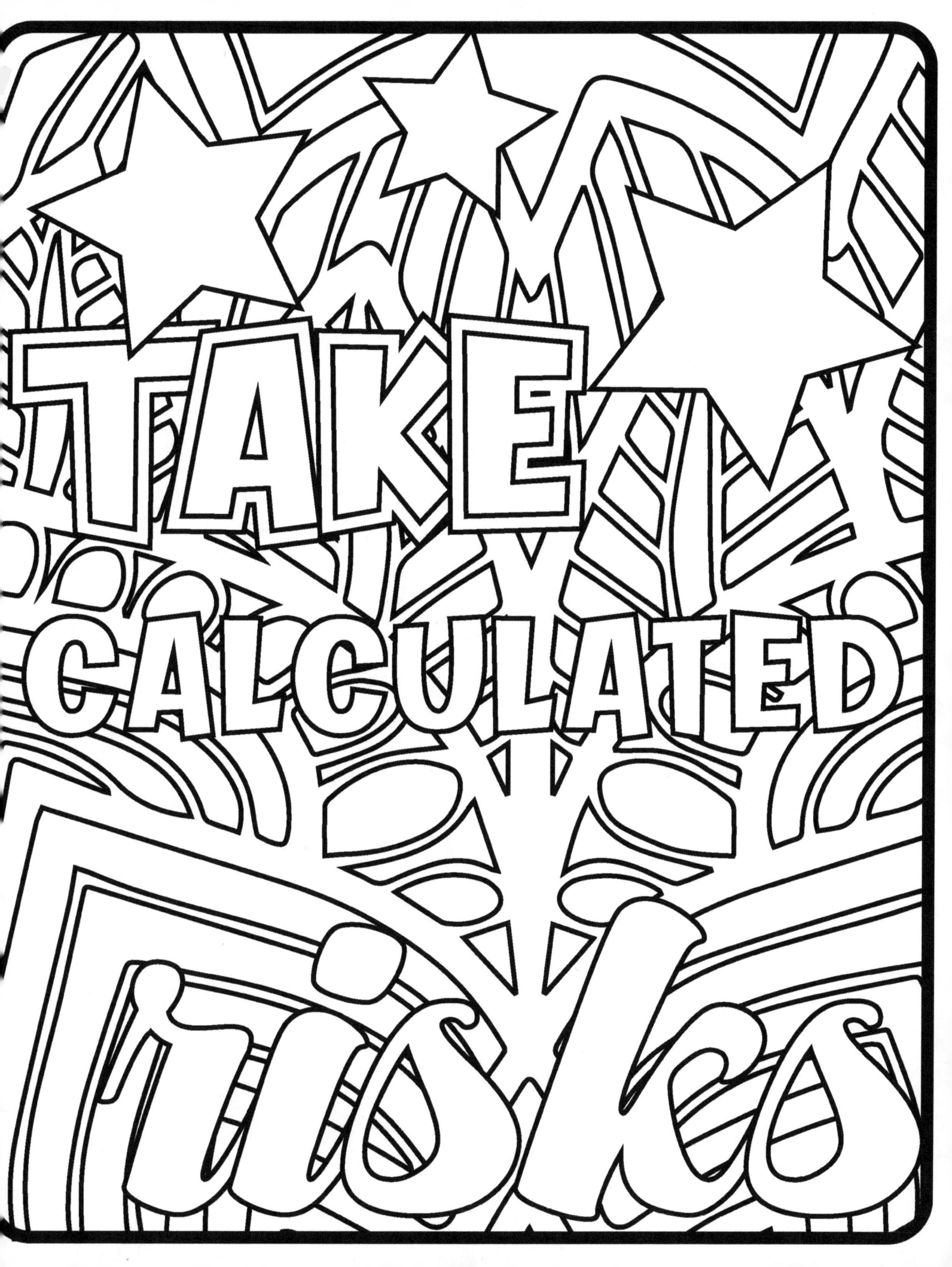

TAKE CALCULATED risks

OVER
THINKER

me?

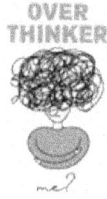

Catherine Worren

We always love to offer free books to our readers.

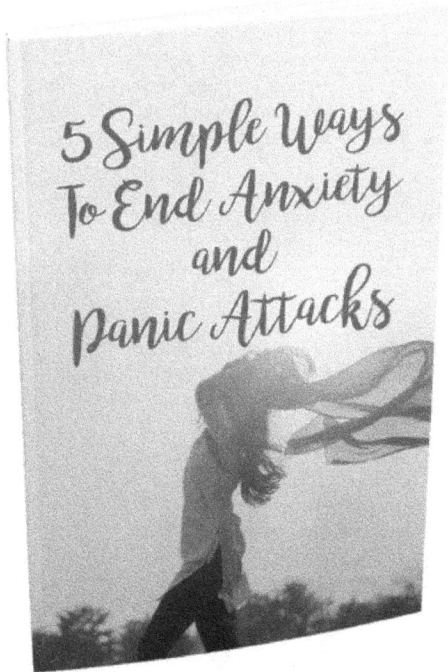

5 Simple Ways
To End Anxiety
and
Panic Attacks

Get your free book by scanning the **QR** code or by sending an email to the address bellow.

✉ Catherine.Worren@yahoo.com

www.ingramcontent.com/pod-product-compliance
Lightning Source LLC
Chambersburg PA
CBHW052117020426
42335CB00021B/2807